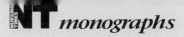

Changing practice: The theory

Anne Mulhall, PhD, MSc, BSc

'The nurses on the ground think that it might be another imposition on them from above, because of all the changes that are going on in the NHS at the moment. I think that is why nurses are suspicious of anything.' This quote, reported in a recent study that investigated the restraints to research-based practice (le May et al, 1998) neatly encapsulates many health care professionals' feelings about change. Throughout the past 10 years a succession of policy initiatives has radically reorganised the way care is delivered (Department of Health and Social Security, 1984; Department of Health, 1989; 1992; 1997). As a result nurses, midwives and health visitors have witnessed a series of seemingly endless changes not only the way in which services are delivered, but also the entire culture of the national health system. Set within this culture of constant, and indeed threatening, change, nurses and other health care workers have, nonetheless, to fashion their own ideas and strategies concerning change in practice. But who decides what should change? How should change be achieved? Should practice change at all? Given the prolific literature on the subject it is difficult to undertake a systematic and comprehensive review of this field of study. Instead this monograph will focus on sifting information that has potential for nursing. To that end we will inspect various theories concerning change, but at the same time examine the 'currency' which these have for the realities of everyday practice.

Theories and models of change

Although the literature on change is replete with different models of change, Egan (1985) makes the useful distinction between explanatory models that describe change in a theoretical way and working models that form the framework for practical action.

Working models tell us how to make changes happen, and this monograph will focus on these.

A distinction is also often made between top-down and bottom-up change although, in practice, it may be difficult to make such a clear distinction.

Top-down approaches

The top-down approach is, not surprisingly, one that features in many management texts. It is exemplified by the organisational development school of thought (Beckhard and Harris, 1987; Plant, 1987).

Organisational development, in terms of health care, has been defined as 'an effort (1), planned, (2) organisation-wide and (3) managed from the top to (4) increase organisational effectiveness and health through (5) planned interventions' (Beckhard, 1969).

Using this approach, managers assess the current demands for change — perhaps from consumers or the government. They then determine how far their organisation matches up to these new demands, the changes that will be required, and the readiness and capacity of the organisation to achieve them. An appropriate plan of action is then devised.

This model of change management is referred to as rational-linear because it assumes that the process of change proceeds through a simple step-by-step unidirectional progression from one stage to the next. Its basis is found in scientific thinking and it rests on the assumption that the social world and the people in it are rational and logical.

The organisational development approach has strongly influenced management theory in the UK and, as a result of the introduction of general management into the NHS, this type of model has increasingly been applied in health care settings (Spurgeon and Barwell, 1991). Upton and Brooks (1995) have provided a very practical guide to using this approach.

Not only is this model used by general managers in the NHS; Wilson (1992) illustrated how the nursing management of a large Canadian hospital was strongly based on an organisational development perspective.

The organisational development model is founded in the work of Lewin, who proposed that change occurred through a three-phase model similar to that described above. Lewin (1951) contended that situations were held in equilibrium and change occurred as a result of driving or resisting forces — the force-field theory of change.

For change to occur, the current state must be 'unfrozen' by people becoming aware of a problem and the necessity for change. Then the forces holding the change in equilibrium must be worked on by increasing the forces driving the change and minimising those resisting it. Finally, everything must be 'refrozen', with the change integrated into the person, the organisation and the culture. This is the most widely known model of planned change, although Spurgeon and Barwell (1991) described several other versions.

The organisational development model was criticised by Pettigrew (1985) who contended that change did not occur as an isolated event but was embedded in a historical, cultural and political background. He argued that change did not occur through a prescriptive intervention plan.

Instead, Pettigrew's research at ICI suggested that change occurred as a result of the conflation between external pressures on the organisation and internal struggles for power, status and reward. Change occurred not through a rational process of managerial planning and goal-setting but as the outcome of power struggles between different interested parties. In this model, change is achieved not through strategic planning but through the delegitimisation of opponents' ideas by building support in the political and cultural systems of the organisation.

Another example of change that does not accord with the prescriptive model was provided by Bennett and Ferlie (1994). Based on empirical case study data from a number of district health authorities the authors demonstrated that the organisational and managerial response to HIV/AIDS 'suggests a much messier, inchoate and emergent innovation process than [that] contained within many of the prescriptive management of change models'.

Bottom-up approaches

The top-down approach to change tends to be based on scientific thinking, rationality and logic. It is based on ideas of leadership and 'change agents' — people usually in positions of power and sometimes from outside the organisation — who 'drive' the change through.

In contrast, bottom-up change is conceptualised as participative. It mirrors some of the characteristics of organic organisations, namely group consensus about decisions, solutions that are sought jointly, high participation, high dependence on the group and the sharing of satisfaction among the group (Plant, 1987).

Participative change can occur only where the power to make decisions is equally shared among staff. Ford and Walsh (1994) suggest that in the bottom-up approach 'efforts should be directed towards team-building and cooperation, as this will maximise flexibility and minimise conflict while supporting individuals, within a supportive team environment, to give of their best'.

Changing practice:
The theory

···

Anne Mulhall

PhD, MSc, BSc

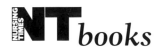

NT *books*

Emap Healthcare Ltd
Greater London House
Hampstead Road
London NW1 7EJ

Nursing Times Clinical Monographs are authoritative, concise, single subject publications designed to provide a critical review of material that will be of value to practising nurses, midwives and health visitors. Their authors, all experts in their field, are asked to be challenging and thought-provoking and to stimulate reflection on current practice. *Nursing Times* Clinical Monographs do not seek to be exhaustive reviews but up-to-date overviews; their critical and evaluative nature is designed to promote best practice through consideration of current evidence.

Topics for publication are decided by the editorial advisory board, with input from practitioners. Monographs are then commissioned as near as possible to the publication date to ensure that the information they contain is the latest available. All manuscripts are reviewed by a board member and a clinician working in the field covered.

Every three months, 12–15 new monographs will be published. They will cover subjects suggested by practitioners (see bottom of page) and any major new developments in the field of nursing care. Each publication will be on sale for a limited time, after which it will be withdrawn and, if necessary, replaced with an updated version.

Suggestions for future titles are welcome and should be sent to Simon Seljeflot at NT Books, Emap Healthcare, Greater London House, London NW1 7EJ

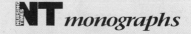

These ideas have resonance with two areas which nursing is increasingly engaging with — critical theory and feminism.

Critical theory and feminism

Critical theory contends that society is structured by meanings, rules and habits that are adhered to by social beings (Allen et al, 1986). The task for critical theorists is to unmask those aspects of society that restrict or limit human freedom by maintaining the status quo. We can do this only by critically reflecting on things we normally take for granted — those rules and traditions that uphold the way we think and go about nursing work. Critical theory may find a use in participative change through two channels (Mulhall, 1998).

First, nursing as a subordinated group in the NHS is forced to take on the characteristics and/or agendas of more dominant groups (doctors or general managers). A knowledge of the basic premise of critical theory will alert nurses to this and the effect it may have on their efforts to introduce change.

The subtle ways in which the power distribution within the NHS works need to be unearthed. For example, if through pressure of workload nurses are unable to be released to sit on important decision-making bodies, or if they have not been equipped with the appropriate skills to function effectively on such bodies, their voices will not be heard. Through critical reflection nursing will be able to expose those social structures that maintain things as they are and thus come to a more insightful analysis of how change might be effected.

Like critical theory, feminism aims to emancipate the oppressed from ideology, the focus here being on gender. Quite obviously, a concern with gender is crucial to the nursing professions, since the majority of nurses are female and, what is more, they espouse a classically 'feminine' attribute — caring. It is important, therefore, for nursing to become more aware of how gender issues affect the construction of social reality, because this is the back-

drop against which change will have to be effected.

What is change, and can it be managed?

Conceptualising change

Although change seems a familiar concept, it is worth considering exactly what we mean when we talk about change. Change as a noun is something that has happened, but here we are more concerned with change as a verb — how changes in practice might be attained more effectively, namely the process of change. However, it is important to reflect on when a change ceases to be one.

For Lewin (1951) this stage occurs when the situation becomes 'refrozen' and the change is integrated into normal practice. Although theoretically this appears sound, in practice it may be quite difficult to ascertain when a change has become fully integrated. This underlines the importance of evaluating changes to determine how far they have become embedded in everyday thinking and practice — in other words, normalised.

What is more, changes may 'revert'. For example, by undertaking a second long-term evaluation of the changes a series of research utilisation workshops have engendered it has been revealed that, although practitioners initially gained skills (such as being able to critically appraise research evidence), these could be rapidly lost once participants had returned to the demands of their daily work and were unable to practise their newly acquired talents (le May et al, 1998).

Moreover, although some changes may be discrete 'revolutionary' events, much change goes on all the time, in a more incremental manner — a sort of evolutionary process. Even the substantial reorganisations of the NHS in the past decade are considered by some to represent an evolutionary series of developments rather than a precipitate change in direction (Spurgeon and Barwell, 1991).

Western ways of viewing the world set great store on moving forward,

Notes

developing, changing. Individualism is highly prized, and personal control and accountability are the goals to strive for. Many management texts echo this theme in their enthusiastic adoption of strategies for planning and leading an organisation or team to a better future. Seen in this light, change ceases to become a morally neutral category, because it personifies progress towards a greater good.

Thus, in Western cultures those who create barriers to change are often perceived as holding up the natural order of things, and resistance to change becomes morally unacceptable. This is perfectly illustrated in some of the labels, such as 'laggard', given in theoretical change models to those who resist change until the last possible moment (Rogers, 1983).

Managing change

Timpson (1996), in her discussion of managing successful change with respect to human resources, stated that the concepts involved were 'as complex as they are contentious, with arguments and counter-arguments espoused weekly in the seemingly ever-growing plethora of literature available'. This emphasises the difficulties in trying to answer the question of whether change can be managed.

Indeed, perhaps before this question can be answered, we need to explore in closer detail what happens when change is proposed, and whether change is universal in nature. Can theories that have been developed in commerce be generalised to the NHS?

What happens when change is proposed?

Although we may hold our own particular attitudes and beliefs we are shaped by our prevailing culture. The culture of nursing provides us with a system of shared ideas, concepts, rules and meanings that not only tell us how to view the world but also inform us how to act in it.

Change may challenge these norms and call into question beliefs, attitudes and practices. It may alter the social balance of power, challenge the way we perceive things, call into question our professional skills, modify our relationships with colleagues and patients or change the entire nature of our work. It is not surprising, then, that change is often viewed as perilous, because it does pose a threat to the normal balance of things.

Furthermore, change affects everyone and everything. In the NHS change may challenge individual professionals, individual patients and their relatives, groups of professionals or the social structure of health care organisations.

For instance, the drive towards evidence-based practice may threaten individual practitioners. Some patients may also be highly resistant to proposed changes — they may be perfectly satisfied with the service they are currently receiving.

Professional groups may be affected. For example, changes in the system for nurse education may be viewed as threatening by nurses who underwent more 'traditional' courses (Maben, 1998).

Change in an organisation may also create a different environment, ethos, or organisational identity — witness the trauma caused by the various amalgamations of London teaching hospitals. This change not only threatened access to services in different localities but also dug more deeply at traditional allegiances held by both professionals and recipients of health care.

A number of models of what happens during the process of change have been derived from early sociological research in the field of agriculture, although this work has been corroborated in doctors (Coleman et al, 1959). The best known model — one which Stocking (1992) discusses in her paper on promoting change in clinical care — is the social interaction and diffusion model based on the work of Rogers and Shoemaker (1971).

This model describes the process involved when an innovation is communicated to the members of a social system. Rogers and Shoemaker proposed that four factors influenced whether 'innovations' (or changes) were accepted and incorporated into practice:

- The relative advantage of a new practice — for instance, how it improves on existing practice;
- How compatible the change is with present practices and staff attitudes;
- The complexity of the innovation — the feasibility for easily understanding and implementing it;
- The possibility that innovations can be tried out, perhaps in a demonstration area.

Innovations that demonstrate high relative advantage and compatibility, lack complexity and can be tried out are more likely to be adopted than changes that do not demonstrate these characteristics.

Rogers (1983) also characterised people in terms of the alacrity with which they took up new changes. Innovators are the first group — those who are willing to take risks — followed by 'early adopters' or opinion leaders who accept the change, which then spreads rapidly via the majority, until it finally reaches the 'laggards'. However, while widely cited, this model has been criticised for failing to appreciate the problems of making change in social systems (Havelock and Havelock, 1973).

Rogers (1983) observed that the factors influencing whether change was adopted largely revolved around the perceptions of those who were involved in introducing the innovation.

It seems clear that the optimum approach to capture such perceptions will be through naturalistic/interpretive research. Such approaches have been used in several nursing studies that have explored the perceptions of those who are involved in change. For example, using grounded theory — an inductive research strategy for generating and confirming theory from data collected in the field — Knight (1998) explored the lived experience of change during a period of curriculum and educational reform in a department of nurse education.

Among other findings, Knight highlighted the grief responses associated with change. Some of the themes that emerged from his data included 'isola-tion', 'alienation' and 'loss'. These data complement similar findings in staff nurses undergoing change, reported by Schoolfield and Orduna (1994), and are consistent with the early stages of grief responses to change outlined by Perlman and Takacs (1990).

Interestingly Knight also commented that differences in response to change between 'movers' and 'waiters' might not reflect a difference in attitude to change but merely related to a slower progression through the same cycle.

A similar study of change in nursing has explored the way in which the introduction of Project 2000 was experienced by nurse managers (Hallett, 1997). Such studies provide significant insight into the process of change and the meaning it has for people. Moreover, researchers using the interpretive paradigm purport to undertake research with rather than on people, an approach that should lend itself to a rich and sustainable understanding of peoples' attitudes and perceptions to change.

Is the NHS different?

Much of the theory and practice of change has evolved from the study of profit-making organisations. Despite the introduction of a general management function and the move towards a market economy, several commentators have argued that the NHS cannot be equated with the more general world of commerce. The goal of the latter is to maximise profit and market share.

In the NHS increased activity will result in increased costs to public spending, which cannot be sustained. Moreover, the provider-consumer relationship in the NHS is unlike that in the high street — on the whole patients do not shop around for their health care needs. They are constrained by the contracts that have been drawn up locally.

Gunn (1989) argued that managers in the NHS must juggle the needs of central and local government alongside the general public interest for an equitable, consistent and accessible service. Furthermore, they must maintain a balance between changes aspired to by clinicians and the needs to meet external political and financial pressures. Thus factors that may drive change in the private sector may not be present in the NHS, and it is important to consider this when exploring strategies to introduce new practices in health care settings.

Making change happen in the NHS

Despite the proliferation of literature on change management, almost all of us could cite examples of changes that have been badly managed. The experiences of a chief officer of a community health council negotiating with a regional health authority provide some ironic, but sadly accurate examples, such as: 'Do not explain immediately, openly, and clearly what you want to do and why. In particular do not admit that the changes proposed have anything to do with resource distribution or cuts' (Pattison, 1996). Nevertheless, change is an integral part of both our professional and private lives. What is needed is a more realistic and sensitive notion of what change is, how it manifests itself,

who is affected, and how we can optimise its challenge.

This would be facilitated by more insightful and open reporting of change initiatives. A good example of this was provided by Dunn (1998) in her discussion of a project in the PACE series (Table 1 below), which sought to bring together staff from primary and secondary settings to bring about enduring and consistent changes in the care of people with leg ulcers.

The author commented that, although theory would advocatee involving all stakeholders in the process, in practice this was difficult. The people who needed to be involved were very preoccupied with giving direct clinical care and meetings had to be frequently reorganised to meet service demands.

Top-down changes are often wrought by managers responding to external financial constraints, governmental directives or even customer dissatisfaction, while bottom-up approaches frequently occur as a result of professional concerns that arise internally. It is important to recognise this distinction because it often affects both the mechanisms put forward to bring about the change and the response to it.

Table 1. Examples of projects aimed at making changes in practice

- PACE: the King's Fund programme on Promoting Action on Clinical Effectiveness. The reports from this pay particular attention to the process of achieving change (for further details see Dunning, 1998; Abi-Aad, 1998; Abi-Aad and Raine, 1998);

- STEP: South Thames Evidence-Based Practice project is a collaborative venture between university departments of health care science, nursing and midwifery, and NHS trusts in the South Thames Region. Nine practice development posts have been established to implement evidence-based practice into a multiprofessional service setting and test its impact, using a clinical audit framework;

- ACE: the Assisting Clinical Effectiveness Programme that aims to foster the implementation of evidence-based practice through clinical guidelines integrated with clinical audit. The ACE programme and the process of change involved has been evaluated by the Centre for Nursing and Midwifery Research, University of Brighton;

- FACTS: the Framework for Appropriate Care Throughout Sheffield project aims to create a reproducible and cost effective framework for changing clinical behaviour. Its efforts have been focused on GP practices (the project web site http://www.shef.ac.uk/uni/projects/facts/ has the full text of the report *Lessons from FACTS*, which gives details of the implications for evidence based change management).

Top-down change

Table 2 below outlines a range of external factors and initiatives that have led to significant changes in professional practice, which are discussed below.

The advent of a general management function and an internal market in the NHS precipitated far-reaching changes in health care practice (Ranade, 1994). The management reforms in particular introduced resource management, made clinical audit compulsory and placed a new emphasis on empowering those who used the service.

The introduction of audit should have a significant effect in terms of changing clinical practice, since its key elements include criteria for good practice, methods for measuring whether these criteria are being met, and mechanisms for implementing appropriate change (Taylor, 1996). As Cheater and Closs (1998) stated, 'the prime purpose of audit is to create change where indicated'.

However, good evidence concerning the effectiveness of audit in bringing about changes in professional practice is scarce (Abi-Aad, 1998). Certainly, a systematic review in the field of continuing medical education reported that audit and feedback were less effective than other change strategies, such as reminders, outreach visits and opinion leaders in changing physicians' performance (Davis et al, 1997).

In contrast, the NHS Executive (1996) quoted several examples of how audit had successfully changed both clinician behaviour and patient outcomes.

Alongside the wholesale reorganisation of the structure and functioning of the NHS other lesser but highly significant policy changes concerning the way care is delivered have occurred. By 1995 clinical effectiveness had been identified as a priority area for the NHS (NHS Executive, 1995), and since then several policy statements and guidance documents have been released (NHS Executive, 1995; 1998).

This increasing emphasis on the provision of effective and efficient health care (Department of Health, 1992; 1997) has neatly dovetailed with the rise of evidence-based practice (Sackett et al, 1997), which aims to integrate 'individual expertise with the best available external evidence from systematic research'.

Evidence-based care is founded on the idea of life-long problem-based learning that leads clinicians to convert their information needs to questions, track down the best evidence, critically appraise this information and then apply the results in practice. If followed, this process will inevitably result in some changes being made as clinicians discover more effective strategies for care.

A more organised and prescriptive route to using evidence in this way is through the development and implementation of guidelines. Guidelines are 'systematically developed statements to assist practitioner and patient decisions about appropriate health care for specific clinical circumstances' (Field and Lohr, 1990).

A recently updated systematic review (Grimshaw et al, 1995) indicated that well-developed, properly disseminated and implemented guidelines that provided strong evidence concerning their recommendations were effective in changing clinical practice.

In comparison, a review by Cheater and Closs (1997) was unable to find sufficiently good evidence to make recommendations concerning the relative effectiveness of methods of dissemination and implementation of

---

Table 2. External factors producing change in clinical practice

- Structural re-organisations of the health service;
- New policy initiatives;
- Changes in ideology;
- Statutory changes in professional responsibility;
- Developments in professional education.

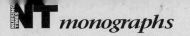

clinical guidelines in nursing. However, the literature they reviewed did indicate that those guidelines that were successfully implemented were introduced in response to clinicians' specific problems and that the support of medical staff was fundamental to successful implementation.

A good synopsis concerning the use of clinical guidelines to develop practice is provided by Seers (1998).

The clinical effectiveness initiative has precipitated a significant number of more local programmes developed either through the NHS strategy for research and development, organisations such as the King's Fund and the royal colleges and charitable bodies. Some examples of relevance to nursing are listed in Table 2.

As new policy is created it may either generate or reflect certain changes in ideology concerning the health service. These ideological changes will also affect clinical practice. For example, there has been a gradual move towards providing a more patient-centred service that meets local needs, is responsive to complaints and sensitive to outcomes that patients as well as professionals consider important (Department of Health, 1989; NHS Executive, 1996).

Statutory changes in the responsibilities of different groups of professionals will also affect changes in the type and extent of the work they do. The introduction of nurse prescribing is a good example of this.

Finally, changes in professional education will change both the nature and expertise of its 'product'. This, in turn, will effect changes in clinical practice. For instance, one of the aims of Project 2000 was to produce nurses capable of reacting to the changing needs of health care who would challenge others and act as agents of change (Maben, 1998).

The changes described so far have usually been conceived and designed by agents external to the NHS workplace. This is not to say that professional health care workers have not been involved but, in general, these initiatives have evoked change by stimulating those in charge of manag-ing health care services to react either to reorganisations of the service and the implications of these policy initiatives and their accompanying changes in ideology or the resource provided by professionals who have gained new skills. These changes have, in general, come top-down.

But as Pattison (1996) noted, 'it is not enough for enthusiastic managers to adopt simple schemata for managing change and then expect other people obediently to pursue the leaders' vision of a better future'. Therefore, although the initiatives discussed have enormous potential for creating change in practice, the stumbling block is often in their implementation.

Perhaps part of the anguish that surrounds much professional change relates to how we frequently feel that such events are out of our hands.

Bottom-up approaches

Perhaps one of the most individualistic and bottom-up approaches to change comes through self-reflection. At an individual level many nurses are beginning to practise reflectively. However, a critical perspective to change must be introduced that incorporates reflective practice in the wider notion of 'conscientisation': nursing must become conscious of itself and the influences on it — how its self has been fashioned through the influence of coercive power relations. This approach to change incorporates not only reflective practice but also dialogue and liberation (Friere, 1994).

In a discussion of being a change agent Boyce (1995) proposed that consciousness preceded individual change and dialogue preceded collective change. Reflective practice involved evaluating and reflecting on the results of her practice before engaging in practice again. However, Boyce contended that this process must also function at an organisational level. Organisations must become 'conscious' of the political, economic, and environmental factors that impinge on them and determine how these filter down through the organisation to affect individuals and groups within it.

At an organisational level reflective

Notes

practice is accomplished through organisational learning. This involves becoming aware of individuals, group processes and systems, constructing alternative actions to move towards shared goals and implementing and evaluating these actions.

As Kendall (1998) noted, 'the health-related literature, particularly that concerning nursing and health promotion, is strewn with references to the concept of empowerment and its relationship to health, healthy living and health care services'.

From the perspective of critical theory (through which it originated) empowerment is perceived as a collective responsibility, although this interpretation has shifted to an emphasis on self-care and self-responsibility evident in much of the literature from the Department of Health (Department of Health, 1990; 1998). Nevertheless, empowerment in its original conception is very much concerned with making changes from the bottom up.

Obviously empowerment conceived in this way may be used in a variety of settings, and several case studies were provided by Kendall (1998).

Tones (1998) emphasised the importance of community participation to health promotion and the integral part it plays in enabling effective changes to occur. However, the extent to which communities are truly involved in decision-making processes concerning health may vary considerably.

Community development represents a fundamentally bottom-up approach to change that encompasses the view that health promotion should 'challenge the culture of contentment to achieve a fairer balance of power and resources in society' (Tones, 1998). Its aim is to enable ordinary people to identify their own needs and have

some say in prioritising, planning, delivering and reviewing services.

This approach to needs assessment is epitomised by the method of rapid appraisal (Rifkin, 1992) that attempts to bring together the perspectives of communities through a dialogue with decision-makers. Its use in the UK is described by Annett and Rifkin (1990), and several projects are described by Ong and Humphris (1994).

Examples of community development in the field of accident prevention are discussed by Roberts (1998). These bottom-up approaches to change through community action will certainly create changes to the practice of health care professionals working in the community. However, they may not accord with the changes the professionals themselves considered important.

Rapid appraisal exercises have highlighted not only the differences in professional and community priorities but also the difference between professionals' perceptions of what the community told them they wanted and the actual view the community held.

Of course, empowerment as a strategy for change may also be used by professionals, and Latter (1998) discussed the case for empowering nurses in the acute setting.

As every nurse knows, small and not so small changes in practice occur every day as they pursue their work, and this has been loosely described in Table 3 below as practice development in the work place (whether that be a hospital ward, a clinic or someone's home).

Examples of such work were provided by James and Smith (in press), who presented four case studies of practice developments based on research. These included the work of the Nursing Research and Practice

---

Table 3. Internal strategies for promoting change in practice

- Reflective practice
- Empowerment
- Practice development in the workplace
- Action research

Notes

Development Unit at St James' and Seacroft University Hospital, Leeds; the development of a nursing strategy for research and development at Bolton Hospitals NHS Trust; the development of nurses' skills in assessment and care-planning that evolved through collaborative work between Guy's and St Thomas' Hospital NHS Trust in London and the Foundation of Nursing Studies; and a project to implement evidence-based practice for the care of patients with leg ulcers undertaken by the primary care and development unit which is part of Waltham Forest Healthcare NHS Trust's primary health care directorate (James and Smith, 1998).

Although these larger initiatives are well-documented, it is impossible to estimate the extent of practice development because the large bulk of such changes go unrecorded in the formal literature. This also reduces the extent of our formal written knowledge concerning those strategies that are most effective in bringing about such changes. Such knowledge may remain local and oral.

It is perhaps important for all nurses to consider mechanisms through which integral or everyday developments and changes could be more effectively disseminated.

Action research is 'a form of self-reflective inquiry undertaken by participants in social situations in order to improve the rationality and justice of their own practices' (Carr and Kemmis, 1986). A number of models have evolved, including the technical collaborative, the mutual collaborative and the enhancement approach (Holter and Schwartz-Barcott, 1993).

Meyer (1995) outlined this evolution from the functionalist perspective through an interpretative phase into a new paradigm that emphasises practitioners as researchers, self-reflection and the development of critical thinking.

All the models include the main characteristics of action research, namely collaboration between researcher and practitioner, identification and resolution of problems, changes in behaviour and theory con-

struction (Newton, 1995). One of the main aims of action research is to create change and improve practice, and much of the current thrust in the field is centred on an essentially bottom-up approach.

The bottom-up and top-down approaches to change are embedded in different world views, and each advocates a different model of achieving change. Bottom-up approaches to change often seem to appeal to health care practitioners who are working directly with patients and clients and, indeed, to patients and clients themselves.

Our experiences tell us that, where people have ownership, change tends to cause less anguish and become more firmly embedded. However, the adoption of such approaches may reflect a more general human desire to gain control over our own destiny, and we need to make sure that this does not cloud our judgment in considering how change might best be effected.

There is no doubt that top-down change is effective. If governmental policy indicates a change in direction concerning the delivery of services then, although they may not 'carry' health care workers or the users of the service with them, such structural if not ideological changes do tend to occur.

Strategies for change may need to use both top-down and bottom-up approaches. Cutliffe and Bassett (1997) used two case study vignettes to illustrate how change theory might be applied in practice. Using the example of introducing research in nursing practice they concluded that there was no one best way of bringing about change and knowledge of several models of change was required.

Conclusion

In practice it is probably quite difficult to separate top-down from bottom-up approaches. Change in practice might encapsulate a conglomerate of different approaches that are not easily teased apart. For example, where does the top start? How do we know if we

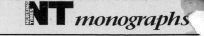

are truly using empowering bottom-up approaches?

Perhaps the issue causing most concern, however, is the dearth of knowledge concerning the effectiveness of particular strategies for change in the field of health care, and whether methods that work in the business world are applicable to the NHS.

Currently many individual projects concerned with achieving changes in clinical practice are being evaluated (Table 2). Furthermore, the Cochrane Effective Practice and Organisation of Care Review Group is working on systematic reviews of educational, behavioural, financial, organisational and regulatory interventions to improve clinical practice. However, such efforts are principally targeted at top-down changes.

The effectiveness of bottom-up change needs to receive similar attention. If practitioners and their managers are to employ a range of approaches to achieving change the effectiveness of all strategies needs to be established. However, such research into effectiveness needs to focus not only on the outcome but also on the process of change and to employ a range of research designs using both quantitative and qualitative methods. **NT**

References

Abi-Aad, G. (1998) Measuring change in the NHS. *Nursing Times*; 94: 43, 58–59.

Abi-Aad, G, Raine, R. (1998) Planning for action. *Nursing Times*; 94: 25; 46.

Allen, D., Benner, P., Diekelmann, N. (1986) Three paradigms for nursing research methodological implications. In: Chinn, P. (ed) *Nursing Research Methodology*. New York: National League for Nursing.

Annett, H., Rifkin, S. (1990) *Improving Urban Health*. Geneva, Switzerland: WHO.

Beckhard, R. (1969) *Organisational Development: Strategies and Models*. Reading, Mass: Addison Wesley.

Beckhard, R., Harris, R.T. (1987) *Organisational Transitions: Managing Complex Change*. Reading, Mass: Addison Wesley.

Bennett, C., Ferlie, E. (1994) *Managing Crisis and Change in Health Care*. Buckingham: Open University Press.

Boyce, M.E. (1995) Solidarity and praxis: being a change agent in a university setting. *Journal of Organisational Change Management;* 8: 6, 58–66.

Carr, W., Kemmis, S. (1986) *Becoming Critical: Education Knowledge and Action Research*. London: Falmer Press.

Cheater, F.M., Closs, S.J. (1998) The relationship between clinical audit and research. In: Roe, B., Webb, C. (eds) *Research and Development in Clinical Nursing Practice*. London: Whurr.

Coleman, J., Katz, E., Menzel, H. (1959) *Medical Innovation: A Diffusion Study*. New York: Bobbs Merrill.

Cutliffe, J.R., Bassett, C. (1997) Introducing change in nursing: the case of research. *Journal of Nursing Management*; 5: 241–247.

Davies, D.A., Thomson, M.A., Oxman, A.D.,

Haynes, R.B. (1997) Changing physician performance: a systematic review of the effect of continuing medical education strategies. *Journal of the American Medical Association* ; 274: 9, 700–705.

Department of Health (1989) *Working for Patients*. London: HMSO.

Department of Health (1990) *The Community Care Act*. London: HMSO.

Department of Health (1992) *The Health of the Nation: A Strategy for Health in England*. London: HMSO.

Department of Health (1997) *The New NHS: Modern, Dependable*. London: HMSO.

Department of Health (1998) *Our Healthier Nation*. London: Stationery Office.

Department of Health and Social Security (1984) *Health Service Management: Implementation of the NHS Management Inquiry Report. HC(84)13*. London: DHSS.

Dunn, C. (1998) Clinically effective leg ulcer care. Nursing Times; 94: 47, 61–63.

Egan, G. (1985) *Change Agent Skills in Helping and Human Settings*. Baltimore, Md: Brooks Cole.

Field, M.J., Lohr, K.N. (1990) *Clinical Practice Guidelines. A Direction of a New Agency*. Washington: Institute of Medicine.

Ford, P., Walsh, M. (1994) *New Rituals for Old. Nursing Through the Looking Glass*. Oxford: Butterworth Heinemann.

Friere, P. (1994) *Pedagogy of the Oppresse*d. New York: Continuum.

Grimshaw, J., Freemantle, N., Wallace, S. et al (1995) Developing and implementing clinical practice guidelines. *Quality in Health Care*; 4: 1, 55–64.

Gunn, L. (1989) A public management approach to the NHS. *Health Services Management Research*; 2: 1, 10–19.

Notes

Hallett, C. (1997) Managing change in nurse education: the introduction of Project 2000 in the community. *Journal of Advanced Nursing*; 25: 4, 836–843.

Havelock, R. G., Havelock, M. (1973) *Training for Change Agents*. Ann Arbor, Mi: University of Michigan Ann Arbor Centre for Research on Utilisation of Scientific Knowledge, Institute for Social Research.

Holter, I.M., Schwartz-Barcott, D. (1993) Action research: what is it? How has it been used and how can it be used in nursing? *Journal of Advanced Nursing*; 18: 2, 298–304.

James, T., Smith, P. (in press) Implementing research: the practice In: Mulhall, A., le May, A. (eds) *Nursing Research: Dissemination and Implementation*. Edinburgh: Churchill Livingstone.

Kendall, K. (ed) (1998) *Health and Empowerment*. London: Arnold.

Knight, S. (1998) A study of the lived experience of change during a period of curriculum and organisational reform in a department of nurse education. *Journal of Advanced Nursing*; 27: 6, 1287–1295.

Latter, S. (1998) Health promotion in the acute setting: the case for empowering nurses. In: Kendall, K. (ed) (1998) *Health and Empowerment*. London: Arnold.

le May, A., Mulhall, A., Alexander, C. (1998) Bridging the research practice gap: exploring the research cultures of practitioners and managers. *Journal of Advanced Nursing*; 28: 2, 428–437.

le May, A., Mulhall, A., Alexander, C., Thornton, C. (1998) Evidence into practice: assessing the impact of a series of national workshops. Durham: Nurse Education Tomorrow International Participative Conference.

Lewin, K. (1951) *Field Theory in the Social Sciences*. New York: Harper.

Maben, J. (in press) Research dissemination and implementation: the role of education. In: Mulhall, A., le May, A. (eds) *Nursing Research: Dissemination and Implementation*. Edinburgh: Churchill Livingstone.

Meyer, J. (1995) Stages in the process: a personal account. *Nurse Researcher*; 2: 3, 24–37.

Mulhall, A. (in press) Creating change in practice. In: Mulhall, A., le May, A. (eds) *Nursing Research: Dissemination and Implementation*. Edinburgh: Churchill Livingstone.

Newton, C.A. (1995) Action research: application in practice. *Nurse Researcher*; 2: 3, 60–71.

NHS Executive (1995) *Improving the Effectiveness of Clinical Services. EL(95)105*. Leeds: NHSE.

NHS Executive (1996) *Promoting Clinical Effectiveness. A Framework for Action in and through the NHS*. Leeds: NHSE.

NHS Executive (1998) *Achieving Effective Practice: A Clinical Effectiveness and Research Information Pack for Nurses, Midwives and Health Visitors*. Leeds: NHSE.

Ong, B.N., Humphris, G. (1994) Prioritising needs with communities. Rapid appraisal methodologies in health. In: Popay, J., Williams, G. (eds) *Researching the People's Health*. London: Routledge.

Pattison, S. (1996) Change management in the British national health service: A worm's eye critique. *Health Care Analysis*; 4: 3, 252–258.

Perlman, D., Takacs, G.T. (1990) The 10 stages of change. *Nursing Management*; 21: 4, 33–38.

Pettigrew, A.M. (1985) *The Awakening Giant: Contingency and Change in ICI*. London: Blackwell.

Plant, R. (1987) *Managing Change and Making it Stick*. London: Fontana.

Ranade, W. (1994) *A Future for the NHS?* London: Longman.

Rifkin, S. (1992) Rapid appraisal for health. *Rapid Rural Appraisal Notes*; 7: 7–12.

Roberts, H. (1998) Empowering communities: the case of childhood accidents. In: Kendall, K. (ed) *Health and Empowerment*. London: Arnold.

Rogers, E.M., Shoemaker, F.F. (1971) *Communication of Innovations: a Cross-Cultural Approach*. New York: Free Press.

Rogers, E.M. (1983) *Diffusion of Innovations*. New York: Free Press.

Sackett, D.L., Richardson, W.S., Rosenberg, W., Haynes, R.B. (1997) *Evidence-Based Medicine. How to Practise and Teach EBM*. Edinburgh: Churchill Livingstone.

Schoolfield, M., Orduna, A. (1994) Understanding staff nurse responses to change: utilisation of a grief-change framework to facilitate innovation. *Clinical Nurse Specialist*; 8: 1, 57–62.

Seers, K. (1998) Use of clinical guidelines in the development of practice. In: Roe, B., Webb, C. (eds) *Research and Development in Clinical Nursing Practice*. London: Whurr.

Spurgeon, P., Barwell, F. (1991) *Implementing Change in the NHS*. London: Chapman and Hall.

Stocking, B. (1992) Promoting change in clinical care. *Quality in Health Care*; 1: 56–60.

Taylor, D. (1996) Quality and professionalism in health care: a review of current initiatives in the NHS. *British Medical Journal*; 312: 7031, 626–629.

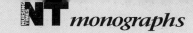

Timpson, J. (1996) Towards an understanding of human resource in the context of change in the NHS: economic sense versus cultural sensibilities? *Journal of Nursing Management*; 4: 6, 315–324.

Tones, K. (1998) Empowerment for health: the challenge. In: Kendall, K. (ed) *Health and Empowerment*. London: Arnold.

Upton, T., Brooks, B. (1995) *Managing Change for the NHS*. London: Kogan Page.

Wilson, D. (1992) Paradigms and nursing management: analysis of the current organisational structure in a large hospital. *Healthcare Management Forum*; 5: 2, 4–9.

Notes

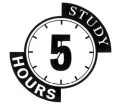

Notes